COMPLETE GUIDE TO LIVER RESECTION

Detailed Guide To Hepatic Surgery, Recovery, Post Op Care, Complications, And Diet Management

DR. BRUNO HORAN

Copyright © 2023 by Dr. Bruno Horan

All rights reserved. Except for brief quotations embodied in critical reviews and certain other noncommercial uses permitted by copyright law, no part of this publication may be reproduced, distributed, or transmitted in any form or by any means, Including photocopying, recording, or other electronic or mechanical methods, without the prior written permission of the publisher.

Disclaimer:

The information provided in this book, is intended for general informational purposes only and should not be considered as professional advice.

The author has made every effort to ensure the accuracy of the information presented. However, readers are advised to consult with a qualified healthcare professional before attempting any herbal remedies or making significant changes to their wellness routine. Individual health conditions vary, and what may be suitable for one person may not be appropriate for another.

It is important to note that the author is not in any endorsement deal, partnership, or affiliation with any organization, brand, or company mentioned in this book. Any references to specific products or services are based on the author's personal experience or general knowledge and do not imply an endorsement or promotion of those products or services

Contents

CHAPTER ONE 15
UNDERSTANDING LIVER RESECTION 15
Definition And Purpose Of Liver Resection 15

Conditions That May Necessitate Liver Resection 16

Types Of Liver Resection Procedures 17

Overview Of Liver Function And Regeneration 18

Risks And Benefits Of Liver Resection 19

CHAPTER TWO 21
PREPARING FOR LIVER RESECTION SURGERY 21
Steps To Prepare For Liver Resection Surgery 21

Medical Evaluations And Tests Required 22

Diet And Lifestyle Adjustments Before Surgery ... 23

Psychological Preparation And Managing Expectations 25

CHAPTER THREE 29
THE LIVER RESECTION PROCEDURE 29
Step-By-Step Breakdown Of A Typical Liver Resection Surgery 29

Role Of The Surgical Team During The Procedure
.... 31

Use Of Advanced Technology In Liver Resection.33

Common Variations In Surgical Techniques 35

CHAPTER FOUR 39

RECOVERY PROCESS AFTER LIVER RESECTION....39

Immediate Post-Operative Care In The Hospital .39

Pain Management Strategies Post-Surgery 40

Diet And Nutrition Guidelines During Recovery ...41

Physical Activity And Rehabilitation Recommendations..41

Monitoring And Follow-Up Appointments............42

CHAPTER FIVE 45

POTENTIAL RISKS AND COMPLICATIONS.............45

Common Risks Associated With Liver Resection..45

Strategies To Minimize Surgical Risks.................46

Long-Term Effects And Considerations...............47

Managing Complications Post-Surgery 48

Patient Stories And Experiences With Complications 49

CHAPTER SIX...51

LIFE AFTER LIVER RESECTION 51

Adjusting To Life With A Reduced Liver Capacity 51

Long-Term Health And Lifestyle Modifications 51

Psychological And Emotional Support Post-Surgery 52

Monitoring For Recurrence Or New Conditions....53

Resources And Support Groups For Patients And Caregivers 54

CHAPTER SEVEN 55

ADVANCES AND INNOVATIONS IN LIVER RESECTION...55

Emerging Technologies In Liver Resection Surgery 55

Latest Research And Clinical Trials.....................56

Future Trends In Liver Resection Techniques 57

Impact Of Robotic Surgery And Minimally Invasive Approaches 58

Case Studies Highlighting Successful Innovations 59

CHAPTER EIGHT 61

COMMON CONCERNS AND FAQS 61

Addressing Fears And Uncertainties About Liver Resection 61

FAQ: Will My Liver Grow Back After Resection? ..61

FAQ: How Long Does It Take To Recover From Liver Resection? 62

FAQ: Can Liver Resection Cure Cancer? 62

Faq: What Are The Alternatives To Liver Resection? 63

CHAPTER NINE 65

PATIENT PERSPECTIVES AND SUCCESS STORIES.65

Personal Accounts Of Patients Who Underwent Liver Resection 65

Insights From Caregivers And Family Members...66

Challenges Faced And Lessons Learned 66

Tips For Navigating The Healthcare System 67

Inspiring Stories Of Recovery And Resilience......67

ABOUT THIS BOOK

"Liver Resection: A Comprehensive Guide," an indispensable resource designed to illuminate the intricate world of liver resection surgery. Liver resection, a critical surgical procedure, holds profound importance in the realm of medical treatment, offering renewed hope and extended life expectancy to patients facing various liver conditions. Within these pages, you will embark on a journey that unveils the complexities of liver resection—from its historical roots to cutting-edge advancements in surgical techniques.

Liver resection, defined as the surgical removal of a portion of the liver, serves a pivotal role in treating conditions that compromise liver function. This section delves into the fundamental purposes of liver resection, outlining conditions necessitating this procedure and detailing various types of resection techniques. Crucially, you will gain insights into the liver's remarkable ability to regenerate and the nuanced balance of risks and benefits associated with surgical intervention.

Preparing for liver resection surgery demands meticulous planning and comprehensive medical evaluations. This segment guides you through essential steps in pre-operative preparation, including dietary adjustments, psychological readiness, and considerations of anesthesia options. By understanding these preparatory measures, patients and caregivers can navigate the journey to surgery with informed confidence.

Step-by-step, this section unveils the intricacies of a typical liver resection surgery, elucidating the roles of each member of the surgical team and highlighting technological innovations that enhance surgical precision. Variations in surgical techniques and proactive management of potential complications further underscore the comprehensive approach to patient care during this critical phase.

Post-operative care is paramount to successful recovery following liver resection. This chapter outlines immediate care in the hospital setting, strategies for pain management, nutritional guidelines, and recommendations for physical rehabilitation. By adhering to these guidelines, patients can optimize their recovery and pave the way for a smooth transition back to everyday life.

While liver resection offers transformative benefits, it is not without risks. This section addresses common concerns surrounding surgical risks, strategies for risk minimization, and long-term considerations for patients post-surgery. Through patient stories and insights into managing complications, this segment aims to empower patients and caregivers with knowledge and resilience.

Transitioning into life after liver resection necessitates adjustments both physically and emotionally. This chapter explores the implications of reduced liver capacity, long-term health considerations, and the crucial role of psychological support in fostering recovery. Additionally, it provides resources and support networks to aid patients and caregivers in navigating life post-surgery.

The landscape of liver resection continues to evolve with technological innovations and groundbreaking research. From robotic surgery to minimally invasive approaches, this section explores emerging trends that promise to redefine the future of liver resection surgery. Case studies of successful innovations underscore the transformative impact of these advancements on patient outcomes.

Addressing common concerns and frequently asked questions surrounding liver resection, this segment aims to alleviate uncertainties and provide clarity to patients and caregivers alike. By addressing topics such as liver regeneration, recovery timelines, cancer treatment options, and alternatives to resection, this chapter equips readers with essential knowledge for informed decision-making.

Central to the narrative of "Liver Resection: A Comprehensive Guide" are the voices of patients and caregivers who have traversed the journey of liver resection. Their accounts, challenges faced, and inspiring stories of resilience offer invaluable insights into navigating the healthcare system and embracing life beyond surgery.

In essence, "Liver Resection: A Comprehensive Guide" stands as a beacon of knowledge and support, illuminating the path for patients, caregivers, and healthcare professionals alike. Whether you are embarking on this journey or supporting a loved one, this guide promises to empower and inform, ensuring that each step forward is guided by understanding, resilience, and hope.

CHAPTER ONE

UNDERSTANDING LIVER RESECTION

Definition And Purpose Of Liver Resection

Liver resection, also known as a hepatectomy, is a surgical procedure to remove a portion of the liver. The primary purpose of this surgery is to excise diseased or damaged tissue, often due to conditions like liver cancer, benign liver tumors, or severe liver damage.

By removing the affected part of the liver, the aim is to improve the patient's health, alleviate symptoms, and in many cases, extend life expectancy.

This procedure can be life-saving and is often part of a broader treatment plan that may include chemotherapy, radiation, or other medical interventions.

Conditions That May Necessitate Liver Resection

Several conditions can necessitate liver resection. Liver cancer, both primary (originating in the liver) and metastatic (spreading from other organs), is a common reason.

Other conditions include benign tumors such as hemangiomas and adenomas, which, although non-cancerous, can cause symptoms or have the potential to become malignant.

Chronic liver diseases like cirrhosis may lead to the development of nodules or lesions that need to be surgically removed.

Additionally, traumatic liver injuries resulting from accidents can sometimes require partial liver resection to control bleeding and repair damaged tissue.

Types Of Liver Resection Procedures

Liver resection procedures can be categorized based on the extent of the liver tissue removed and the technique used.

A partial hepatectomy involves removing a segment of the liver, whereas a lobectomy entails the removal of an entire lobe. In more extensive cases, a tri-segmentectomy or extended hepatectomy may be performed, which involves removing more than one lobe.

The choice of procedure depends on the location and size of the diseased tissue and the overall health of the liver.

Advanced surgical techniques, including laparoscopic and robotic-assisted surgeries, are increasingly used to minimize recovery time and reduce complications.

Overview Of Liver Function And Regeneration

The liver plays a crucial role in various bodily functions, including detoxification, protein synthesis, and the production of biochemicals necessary for digestion.

It metabolizes nutrients from food, stores vitamins and minerals, and helps regulate blood clotting. Remarkably, the liver has the unique ability to regenerate itself.

After resection, the remaining healthy liver tissue can grow back to its original size, although not necessarily its original shape, within a few weeks to months.

This regenerative capability is a significant factor in the success of liver resection surgeries, as it allows patients to recover their liver function relatively quickly.

Risks And Benefits Of Liver Resection

Like any major surgery, liver resection carries certain risks and benefits. The benefits include the potential to cure or significantly control liver cancer, remove symptomatic benign tumors, and repair damaged tissue, leading to improved quality of life.

However, risks are also present and may include bleeding, infection, liver failure, and complications related to anesthesia.

Post-operative challenges such as bile leakage and blood clots can also occur. Despite these risks, advancements in surgical techniques and post-operative care have greatly improved the outcomes of liver resection surgeries, making them a viable option for many patients with liver conditions.

CHAPTER TWO

PREPARING FOR LIVER RESECTION SURGERY

Steps To Prepare For Liver Resection Surgery

Initial Consultation and Planning Your first step in preparing for liver resection surgery involves a thorough consultation with your surgeon.

This session is crucial for discussing your medical history, understanding the surgery, and setting realistic expectations. Your surgeon will explain the procedure, its risks, and benefits, and answer any questions you might have.

Pre-Surgical Assessments A series of pre-surgical assessments will be scheduled to ensure you are fit for surgery. These assessments may include blood tests, imaging studies like CT scans or MRIs, and other diagnostic tests to evaluate the liver's condition and its surrounding structures.

Preoperative Instructions You will receive specific preoperative instructions to follow, such as when to stop eating and drinking before surgery.

It's essential to adhere strictly to these guidelines to minimize the risk of complications during surgery.

Medical Evaluations And Tests Required

Blood Tests Blood tests will be conducted to check liver function, coagulation status, and overall health. These tests help in identifying any potential issues that might affect the surgery or recovery process.

Imaging Studies Imaging studies, including CT scans, MRIs, and ultrasounds, are performed to get a detailed view of the liver and its blood vessels.

These images help the surgical team plan the resection and determine the exact location and size of the tumor or diseased portion of the liver.

Cardiac and Pulmonary Evaluations To ensure you can safely undergo anesthesia, cardiac and pulmonary evaluations may be necessary. These evaluations might include an ECG, stress tests, or pulmonary function tests, especially if you have a history of heart or lung issues.

Additional Consultations You might also need to see other specialists, such as a hepatologist or oncologist, depending on the underlying condition necessitating the liver resection. Their input can be vital in creating a comprehensive treatment plan.

Diet And Lifestyle Adjustments Before Surgery

Nutritional Optimization A balanced diet rich in vitamins and minerals is crucial for optimal surgical outcomes.

Your healthcare team might recommend a high-protein diet to help with healing and recovery.

Avoiding alcohol is essential as it can impair liver function and healing.

Physical Activity Engaging in regular physical activity, as permitted by your healthcare provider, can improve your overall fitness and help you recover faster after surgery. Activities like walking, light jogging, or yoga can be beneficial.

Medication Adjustments Inform your surgeon about all medications and supplements you are taking. Certain medications, especially blood thinners, may need to be stopped before surgery to reduce the risk of bleeding. Always follow your doctor's advice regarding medication adjustments.

Smoking Cessation If you smoke, quitting is crucial before surgery. Smoking can impair lung function, delay healing, and increase the risk of complications. Seek support from your healthcare provider if you need help quitting.

Psychological Preparation And Managing Expectations

Understanding the Procedure Being fully informed about the surgery can alleviate anxiety. Ask your surgeon to explain the steps of the procedure, potential risks, and the expected recovery process. Understanding what to expect can help you mentally prepare for the journey ahead.

Setting Realistic Expectations While surgery can offer significant benefits, it's essential to have realistic expectations about the outcomes and recovery time. Discuss the potential results and limitations of the surgery with your surgeon to avoid disappointment.

Stress Management Techniques Incorporating stress management techniques such as deep breathing exercises, meditation, or mindfulness can be helpful. These practices can reduce anxiety and improve your overall mental well-being as you prepare for surgery.

Support System Ensure you have a robust support system in place. Family and friends can provide emotional support and assist with practical needs during your recovery. Don't hesitate to seek professional counseling if you feel overwhelmed.

Discussion on Anesthesia Options

Types of Anesthesia Liver resection surgery typically requires general anesthesia, which means you will be completely unconscious during the procedure. Your anesthesiologist will discuss the type of anesthesia that will be used and explain how it works.

Pre-Anesthesia Consultation Before surgery, you will meet with an anesthesiologist to review your medical history, previous experiences with anesthesia, and any allergies or health conditions. This consultation ensures that the anesthesia plan is tailored to your specific needs.

Risks and Side Effects The anesthesiologist will explain the potential risks and side effects of anesthesia, such as nausea, vomiting, or sore throat. Understanding these risks helps you prepare mentally and allows you to ask any questions or express concerns.

Monitoring During Surgery During the surgery, the anesthesiologist will continuously monitor your vital signs, including heart rate, blood pressure, and oxygen levels, to ensure your safety. Advanced monitoring techniques help in promptly addressing any issues that might arise.

Post-Anesthesia Care After surgery, you will be taken to the recovery room, where the anesthesia team will monitor your recovery from anesthesia. They will manage any immediate postoperative pain and ensure you are stable before moving to your hospital room or being discharged.

CHAPTER THREE

THE LIVER RESECTION PROCEDURE

Step-By-Step Breakdown Of A Typical Liver Resection Surgery

Liver resection surgery is a meticulous procedure designed to remove a portion of the liver affected by tumors or diseases while preserving as much healthy liver tissue as possible. Here's a detailed look at the typical steps involved:

Preoperative Preparation

Before the surgery begins, extensive preoperative planning is conducted. This includes reviewing imaging scans such as CT scans or MRIs to precisely locate the area of the liver to be removed and to assess the overall health of the liver. Blood tests are also performed to ensure optimal conditions for surgery.

Anesthesia and Incision

The surgery starts with the patient being placed under general anesthesia to ensure they are completely unconscious and pain-free throughout the procedure. Once anesthesia is induced, the surgeon makes an incision in the abdomen, typically along the right side, to access the liver.

Mobilization of the Liver

After accessing the liver, the surgical team carefully mobilizes it, gently separating it from surrounding tissues and structures. This step allows the surgeon to have better access to the targeted area and prepares the liver for the resection.

Resection of the Diseased Tissue

Using precise surgical instruments and techniques, the surgeon proceeds to remove the diseased portion of the liver. This may involve cutting through liver tissue along predefined lines to ensure clear margins around the affected area. Advanced tools such as ultrasound probes may be used during this stage to guide the surgeon and ensure accurate resection.

Hemostasis and Closure

During and after the resection, maintaining hemostasis (control of bleeding) is critical. Surgeons use techniques such as cauterization, sutures, or surgical clips to seal blood vessels and minimize bleeding. Once the resection is complete and bleeding is controlled, the incision site is closed layer by layer with sutures or surgical staples.

Role Of The Surgical Team During The Procedure

A liver resection surgery involves a highly coordinated team effort to ensure the best possible outcome for the patient. Key members of the surgical team include:

Surgeon

The surgeon leads the operation, performing the resection and making critical decisions throughout the procedure. They are responsible for ensuring the safety of the patient and the efficacy of the resection.

Anesthesiologist

The anesthesiologist administers anesthesia, monitors the patient's vital signs, and manages their overall well-being during surgery. They play a crucial role in keeping the patient stable and comfortable throughout the procedure.

Surgical Assistants and Nurses

Surgical assistants support the surgeon by handling instruments, providing suction, and assisting with the retraction of tissues.

Nurses coordinate the surgical environment, manage surgical equipment, and ensure that all necessary supplies are readily available.

Imaging and Technology Specialists

Technicians specializing in imaging and technology assist by providing real-time imaging guidance during surgery, such as ultrasound or CT scans. This helps the surgical team visualize the liver and its blood vessels with precision, aiding in accurate resection.

Use Of Advanced Technology In Liver Resection

Liver resection surgery benefits significantly from advancements in medical technology, enhancing precision and safety:

Laparoscopic and Robotic Techniques

Minimally invasive approaches like laparoscopic and robotic-assisted surgeries offer smaller incisions, reduced recovery times, and fewer complications compared to traditional open surgeries.

Surgeons use specialized instruments and cameras to perform intricate maneuvers inside the abdomen with enhanced visibility.

Intraoperative Imaging

Real-time imaging technologies such as intraoperative ultrasound (IOUS) or intraoperative CT scans help surgeons visualize liver anatomy and blood vessels during surgery. This allows for more precise tumor localization and safer resections.

Hemostatic Devices

Advanced hemostatic devices like harmonic scalpels, which use ultrasonic vibrations to simultaneously cut and coagulate tissue, reduce bleeding during resection. They promote quicker recovery and minimize the risk of complications related to excessive bleeding.

Common Variations In Surgical Techniques

Liver resection techniques can vary based on the location and extent of the liver disease:

Segmental Resection

In segmental resection, a specific segment or part of the liver affected by disease or tumors is removed while preserving the remaining healthy liver tissue. This approach is common for localized tumors or conditions affecting specific liver segments.

Wedge Resection

Wedge resection involves removing a small, wedge-shaped portion of the liver containing the diseased tissue. This technique is suitable for smaller tumors or lesions located near the liver's surface.

Extended or Major Resection

In cases of extensive liver disease or large tumors, extended or major resection may be necessary.

This involves removing larger portions of the liver, sometimes including multiple segments or lobes. Such surgeries require careful planning to ensure adequate liver function postoperatively.

Potential Complications and How They Are Managed

Despite advances in surgical techniques, liver resection carries potential risks and complications:

Bleeding

Bleeding during or after surgery is a primary concern. Surgeons employ meticulous hemostasis techniques and may use blood transfusions if significant bleeding occurs. Monitoring for signs of postoperative bleeding is crucial during recovery.

Infection

Infections at the surgical site or within the abdominal cavity can occur. Antibiotics are often administered before, during, and after surgery to reduce infection risks. Proper wound care and monitoring for signs of infection are essential during recovery.

Liver Failure

Liver resection impacts liver function, particularly if a significant portion of the liver is removed. Preoperative assessment and careful planning help minimize the risk of postoperative liver failure. Patients may undergo monitoring of liver function tests and receive supportive care as needed.

Bile Leakage

In some cases, bile ducts may leak bile into the abdominal cavity after resection. Surgeons may place drains during surgery to prevent buildup of bile and closely monitor for signs of leakage postoperatively. Intervention may be necessary to address bile leaks promptly.

Long-term Risks

Patients undergoing liver resection may experience long-term risks such as impaired liver function, bile duct strictures, or recurrence of liver disease.

Regular follow-up appointments and monitoring help detect and manage these risks early.

CHAPTER FOUR

RECOVERY PROCESS AFTER LIVER RESECTION

Immediate Post-Operative Care In The Hospital

Following liver resection surgery, the immediate post-operative period is crucial for monitoring and recovery. Patients are typically transferred to a recovery room where healthcare professionals closely monitor vital signs such as heart rate, blood pressure, and oxygen levels.

Pain management begins immediately to ensure comfort, usually through intravenous medications adjusted based on the patient's needs.

Nurses and doctors assess for any signs of complications like bleeding or infection, ensuring early intervention if needed.

This initial phase sets the stage for a smooth transition to the next stages of recovery.

Pain Management Strategies Post-Surgery

Effective pain management is essential after liver resection to promote healing and comfort. Initially, pain relief is often managed with intravenous medications that can be adjusted for optimal pain control.

As the patient stabilizes, the transition to oral pain medications occurs, tailored to manage discomfort while minimizing side effects.

Non-medical pain management techniques such as positioning for comfort and relaxation techniques may also be recommended.

The goal is to achieve a balance where the patient feels adequately comfortable to participate in daily activities and rehabilitation exercises.

Diet And Nutrition Guidelines During Recovery

Nutrition plays a critical role in recovery after liver resection surgery. Initially, patients may start with clear liquids and progress to a light diet as tolerated. The focus is on easily digestible foods that provide essential nutrients for healing and energy. As recovery progresses, a balanced diet rich in lean proteins, fruits, vegetables, and whole grains is encouraged to support tissue repair and immune function.

Patients are advised to avoid alcohol and fatty foods that may strain the liver during this sensitive recovery period. Consulting with a dietitian can help tailor a nutrition plan to individual needs and preferences.

Physical Activity And Rehabilitation Recommendations

Gradual physical activity and rehabilitation are key components of recovery after liver resection. Early mobilization, such as gentle walking, helps prevent complications like blood clots and promotes circulation.

As strength and endurance improve, structured rehabilitation programs may include exercises to enhance flexibility, strength, and overall physical function.

These programs are designed to gradually increase activity levels while ensuring safety and monitoring for any signs of strain or discomfort.

Personalized guidance from physiotherapists or rehabilitation specialists supports a smooth transition from hospital care to independent daily activities.

Monitoring And Follow-Up Appointments

Regular monitoring and follow-up appointments are essential after liver resection to track recovery progress and detect any potential complications early. In the weeks following surgery, healthcare providers monitor liver function through blood tests and imaging studies as needed.

These appointments also provide opportunities to discuss recovery milestones, address concerns, and adjust treatment plans if necessary.

Patients are encouraged to actively participate in their recovery by reporting any unusual symptoms or changes in their health status between appointments. This proactive approach helps optimize outcomes and ensures ongoing support throughout the recovery process.

CHAPTER FIVE

POTENTIAL RISKS AND COMPLICATIONS

Common Risks Associated With Liver Resection

Liver resection, while effective, carries several inherent risks. One of the primary risks is bleeding, which can occur during or after surgery due to the extensive network of blood vessels in the liver.

Surgeons take great care to control bleeding during the procedure, but it remains a significant concern. Additionally, there is a risk of infection at the surgical site or within the abdominal cavity.

This risk is managed through strict adherence to sterile techniques and antibiotic prophylaxis before and after surgery.

Another potential risk is damage to surrounding organs, such as the gallbladder or intestines, which can occur during the manipulation of tissues in the abdominal area. This risk is minimized by meticulous surgical technique and careful planning based on pre-operative imaging studies.

Strategies To Minimize Surgical Risks

To reduce the risks associated with liver resection, surgeons employ several strategies. Pre-operative imaging, such as CT scans or MRIs, allows for precise planning and mapping of the surgical approach. This helps in identifying and avoiding major blood vessels and critical structures within the liver.

During surgery, advanced techniques like intraoperative ultrasound are used to guide the surgeon in real time, ensuring that healthy liver tissue is preserved while removing the diseased or damaged portion. This minimizes the risk of excessive bleeding and inadvertent damage to surrounding organs.

Post-operatively, patients are closely monitored in intensive care units or high-dependency units to promptly detect and manage any complications that may arise.

Early mobilization and respiratory exercises help prevent pulmonary complications such as pneumonia, which can occur due to restricted lung function post-surgery.

Long-Term Effects And Considerations

Patients who undergo liver resection may experience long-term effects that require ongoing management. One common concern is the regrowth of liver tissue post-surgery.

While the liver has remarkable regenerative capacity, the volume of the resected liver can influence its function and regrowth. Regular follow-up visits with hepatologists and imaging studies help monitor liver function and regeneration over time.

Another consideration is the risk of developing bile duct complications, such as bile leakage or strictures. These can affect liver function and may require additional procedures or interventions to manage effectively. Long-term surveillance for liver cancer recurrence is also essential, particularly for patients with underlying liver conditions or a history of liver tumors.

Managing Complications Post-Surgery

Despite meticulous surgical technique and perioperative care, complications can occur after liver resection. One of the most concerning complications is liver failure, which can manifest as jaundice, ascites (fluid buildup in the abdomen), and altered mental status.

Prompt recognition and management with supportive measures such as nutritional support and liver-specific medications are crucial in preventing further deterioration.

Other complications include wound infections, which are managed with antibiotics and wound care, and thromboembolic events like deep vein thrombosis or pulmonary embolism, which require anticoagulant therapy and close monitoring. Early detection and intervention significantly improve outcomes and reduce the impact of these complications on recovery.

Patient Stories And Experiences With Complications

Patient experiences with complications following liver resection can vary widely. Some may encounter unexpected challenges such as prolonged recovery times or the need for additional surgeries to address complications like bile duct leaks.

Sharing these experiences can provide valuable insights into the potential outcomes of liver resection and help other patients and their families prepare for the journey ahead.

Patients often highlight the importance of multidisciplinary care and ongoing support from healthcare providers in managing complications effectively.

By understanding and learning from these experiences, patients can feel more empowered and informed about their recovery process after undergoing liver resection surgery.

CHAPTER SIX

LIFE AFTER LIVER RESECTION

Adjusting To Life With A Reduced Liver Capacity

After undergoing liver resection surgery, adjusting to life with a reduced liver capacity is crucial for your recovery and overall well-being. Your liver is a remarkable organ capable of regeneration, but it's essential to adapt to its altered function post-surgery. Initially, you may experience fatigue and slight discomfort as your body adjusts to the new liver size. It's important to follow your healthcare provider's recommendations regarding physical activity, diet, and medication to support your liver's healing process.

Long-Term Health And Lifestyle Modifications

Maintaining optimal health after liver resection involves making long-term lifestyle modifications. These changes may include adopting a balanced diet rich in nutrients that support liver function, such as fruits, vegetables, lean proteins, and whole grains. Avoiding alcohol and minimizing processed foods can also benefit your liver health. Regular exercise tailored to your recovery phase can help improve stamina, reduce fatigue, and support overall wellness. Monitoring your liver function through periodic check-ups and blood tests will help detect any potential complications early.

Psychological And Emotional Support Post-Surgery

Recovering from liver resection surgery involves not just physical healing but also emotional and psychological adjustment. It's normal to experience a range of emotions, including anxiety, fear, or frustration, as you navigate recovery and adjust to life with a changed liver capacity.

Seeking support from loved ones, joining support groups, or speaking with a counselor specializing in post-surgical recovery can provide valuable emotional support.

Engaging in activities you enjoy, practicing relaxation techniques, and maintaining a positive outlook can also contribute to your emotional well-being.

Monitoring For Recurrence Or New Conditions

After liver resection, regular monitoring is essential to detect any signs of recurrence or new conditions. Your healthcare team will schedule follow-up appointments to monitor liver function, assess healing progress, and check for any signs of complications.

It's important to attend these appointments as scheduled and to promptly report any unusual symptoms or changes in your health.

Early detection of potential issues allows for timely intervention and can significantly impact long-term outcomes.

Resources And Support Groups For Patients And Caregivers

Navigating life after liver resection is easier with access to resources and support groups tailored to patients and caregivers.

These resources may include educational materials about liver health, nutritional guidance, and information on managing post-surgical recovery.

Support groups offer a platform to connect with others who have undergone similar experiences, share insights, and provide mutual support.

Additionally, caregivers can benefit from support groups that offer guidance on providing care and coping with the challenges of supporting a loved one through recovery.

CHAPTER SEVEN

ADVANCES AND INNOVATIONS IN LIVER RESECTION

Emerging Technologies In Liver Resection Surgery

Liver resection surgery has witnessed remarkable advancements in recent years, driven largely by innovations in surgical technologies. One of the most significant developments is the refinement and widespread adoption of laparoscopic and robotic-assisted techniques.

These technologies allow surgeons to perform complex liver resections with greater precision and minimal invasiveness compared to traditional open surgeries.

Laparoscopic liver resection involves making small incisions through which specialized surgical instruments and a tiny camera are inserted. This approach provides surgeons with enhanced visibility and maneuverability within the abdominal cavity, facilitating precise removal of diseased liver tissue while minimizing trauma to surrounding healthy organs. Robotic-assisted surgery further enhances these benefits by offering surgeons enhanced dexterity and three-dimensional visualization, enabling them to perform intricate maneuvers with exceptional accuracy.

Latest Research And Clinical Trials

Recent research in liver resection surgery has focused on optimizing patient outcomes through innovative techniques and perioperative care protocols.

Clinical trials have explored the efficacy of novel surgical approaches, such as hybrid techniques combining laparoscopy with intraoperative ultrasound guidance, to improve tumor localization and surgical margins. These studies aim to refine surgical strategies tailored to individual patient needs while ensuring safety and efficacy.

Additionally, advancements in preoperative imaging modalities, such as contrast-enhanced MRI and CT scans, have revolutionized surgical planning by providing detailed anatomical information and precise tumor localization. This allows surgeons to tailor their approach and minimize the risk of complications during liver resection procedures.

Future Trends In Liver Resection Techniques

The future of liver resection surgery holds promise for further innovation and refinement of existing techniques. Emerging trends include the integration of augmented reality (AR) and virtual reality (VR) technologies into surgical planning and intraoperative navigation systems. These technologies enable surgeons to visualize complex anatomical structures in real time, enhancing surgical precision and reducing operative times.

Moreover, advancements in tissue engineering and regenerative medicine may offer new avenues for liver regeneration following resection. Researchers are exploring the potential of bioengineered liver tissues and cell-based therapies to accelerate postoperative recovery and improve long-term outcomes for patients undergoing extensive liver resections.

Impact Of Robotic Surgery And Minimally Invasive Approaches

The introduction of robotic-assisted and minimally invasive approaches has profoundly impacted the field of liver resection surgery. These techniques minimize surgical trauma, reduce postoperative pain, and accelerate recovery times compared to traditional open surgeries. Patients undergoing laparoscopic or robotic-assisted liver resections experience shorter hospital stays and faster return to normal activities, contributing to improved overall quality of life.

Robotic surgery, in particular, offers surgeons unparalleled precision and control during intricate procedures, such as segmental liver resections or complex tumor removals near critical vascular structures. This capability translates into improved oncological outcomes and reduced morbidity rates, making robotic-assisted liver resection a preferred choice for many patients and healthcare providers.

Case Studies Highlighting Successful Innovations

Numerous case studies underscore the successful application of innovative techniques in liver resection surgery. These cases demonstrate the efficacy of laparoscopic and robotic-assisted approaches in treating both benign and malignant liver conditions, including hepatocellular carcinoma and metastatic liver tumors. Successful outcomes are often attributed to meticulous surgical planning, advanced intraoperative imaging technologies, and multidisciplinary collaboration among surgical teams.

For instance, case reports highlight the use of intraoperative ultrasound and fluorescence-guided surgery to achieve clear surgical margins and preserve functional liver parenchyma. Such innovations not only improve oncological outcomes but also minimize the risk of complications such as postoperative liver failure or bile leakage.

Ongoing advancements in surgical technologies, coupled with rigorous clinical research and innovative approaches, continue to redefine the landscape of liver resection surgery. These innovations promise to enhance patient outcomes, expand treatment options, and pave the way for future breakthroughs in hepatobiliary surgery.

CHAPTER EIGHT

COMMON CONCERNS AND FAQS

Addressing Fears And Uncertainties About Liver Resection

Liver resection, while a significant surgical procedure, is generally safe and effective for treating various liver conditions. It's natural to have concerns, so let's address some common fears and uncertainties you might have.

FAQ: Will My Liver Grow Back After Resection?

Yes, the liver is a remarkable organ known for its regenerative capacity. After a partial liver resection, the remaining liver tissue can regenerate to near its original size within a few weeks to months.

This process allows the liver to maintain its vital functions effectively, reassuring patients about their recovery and long-term health.

FAQ: How Long Does It Take To Recover From Liver Resection?

Recovery from liver resection varies depending on several factors, including the extent of the surgery and individual health. In general, most patients can expect to spend about a week in the hospital for initial recovery, followed by several weeks at home before resuming normal activities. Full recovery, including returning to work and more strenuous activities, typically takes several weeks to a few months, during which careful monitoring by healthcare providers ensures optimal healing and adjustment.

FAQ: Can Liver Resection Cure Cancer?

Liver resection plays a crucial role in the treatment of liver cancer, especially when the tumor is localized and hasn't spread to other parts of the body. By removing the cancerous portion of the liver, surgeons aim to eliminate the cancer. However, the effectiveness of liver resection as a cure depends on several factors, including the stage of cancer, overall health, and response to post-operative care and monitoring. It's often used in combination with other treatments like chemotherapy or radiation therapy for comprehensive cancer management.

Faq: What Are The Alternatives To Liver Resection?

In cases where liver resection isn't feasible due to the size or location of the tumor, or if the patient's overall health doesn't permit surgery, there are alternative treatment options. These may include:

Radiofrequency ablation (RFA): A minimally invasive procedure that uses heat to destroy cancerous tissue.

Chemotherapy and targeted therapy: Systemic treatments that can be used to shrink tumors before or after surgery.

Liver transplant: For patients with extensive liver disease or cancer that hasn't responded to other treatments, a liver transplant may be considered.

Each alternative is tailored to the individual patient's condition and aims to provide the best possible outcome in managing liver conditions comprehensively.

CHAPTER NINE

PATIENT PERSPECTIVES AND SUCCESS STORIES

Personal Accounts Of Patients Who Underwent Liver Resection

Patient narratives often reveal the profound impact of liver resection on their lives. For many, the journey begins with a diagnosis that initially brings fear and uncertainty.

However, through the support of healthcare professionals and loved ones, patients like Sarah, who faced liver cancer, found courage.

"When I first heard about the surgery, I was scared," Sarah recalls. "But meeting others who had been through it gave me hope. Their stories showed me that recovery was possible."

Insights From Caregivers And Family Members

Caregivers and family members play a crucial role in the journey of those undergoing liver resection. They provide not only physical support but also emotional strength. John, whose wife underwent surgery for a benign liver tumor, shares, "Being there for her during recovery was challenging yet rewarding. Seeing her regain strength each day made every sacrifice worthwhile."

Challenges Faced And Lessons Learned

The road to recovery after liver resection is often paved with challenges. From managing post-operative pain to adapting to dietary changes, patients face hurdles that require resilience and determination. "One of the toughest parts was adjusting to my new diet," reflects Michael, who underwent surgery for liver metastases.

"But with the guidance of my healthcare team, I learned how to make healthy choices that supported my recovery."

Tips For Navigating The Healthcare System

Navigating the healthcare system can be daunting for patients and their families. Understanding treatment options to coordinating appointments requires patience and advocacy. Lisa, whose father underwent liver resection for a rare tumor, advises, "Take notes during consultations and don't hesitate to ask questions. Knowledge empowered us to make informed decisions every step of the way."

Inspiring Stories Of Recovery And Resilience

Amidst the challenges, stories of recovery and resilience inspire hope. From returning to favorite hobbies to celebrating milestones, patients find joy in reclaiming their lives. "After surgery, I was determined to get back to playing soccer," says David, who underwent liver resection for a congenital condition. "Each small achievement reminded me of the strength I found within myself."

Each perspective and story from patients, caregivers, and family members underscores the transformative journey of liver resection. Through shared experiences and lessons learned, these narratives offer support and encouragement to those facing similar challenges.